C000270046

ORAL SEX

QUIVER

Contents

FOR HIM

FOR HER

INNER PEACE	SULTRY SQUIRTER
THE VOYEUR	FROM THE HART
THE REMOTE CONTROL	THE CRAVING CAPTIVE
TOO GOOD TO BE TRUE	UNDER THE HOOD
TIGHT TWIRL	CUTE AND COMING
OPEN SESAME	SWEET PEACH
BACK DOOR DINING	TONGUE MASTER
THE BREAST MAN	AH, THERE'S THE RUB
MAKE HER PURR	THE KITTY KAT
BEGGING FOR MORE	THE FRENCH KISS
LUSTY LOINS	THE SIZZLE
BOOTYLICIOUS	BOTTOM'S UP
SEXUAL HEARTBEAT	

HOW TO USE THIS BOOK

Oral sex is a sensual, intense indulgence for both men and women that can be enjoyed as a tantalizing opening act or the climactic main event. This book is intended to open up new avenues of exploration for adventurous lovers who are looking to spice up their already red-hot sex lives.

As you flip through, browse The Basics section to get a taste for each technique. If something piques your interest, read on and explore the Blow-by-Blow and Lick-by-Lick sections for a more detailed set of instructions, and tips for heating things up before you get down to business.

With 50 techniques and a number of variations included in all, even the most eager of lovers won't want to try every move in one sitting. I suggest that you experiment with one or two at a time so that you can gauge your partner's reactions, add your personal touch, and perfect your technique. Blindfold your lover and have him pick page from the book each night, or select three moves and let her choose one from your "favorites" list. If you want to build anticipation throughout the day, pick a position first thing in the morning and send a text, reminding them about your "special request," to make sure they get the message. You may even want to take this book on the road to relish in the excitement of sex on-the-go!

As you incorporate them into your erotic routine, you'll be inspired to tweak the moves, make additions, and create a personalized repertoire to take your sex lives to new heights.

FOR HIM

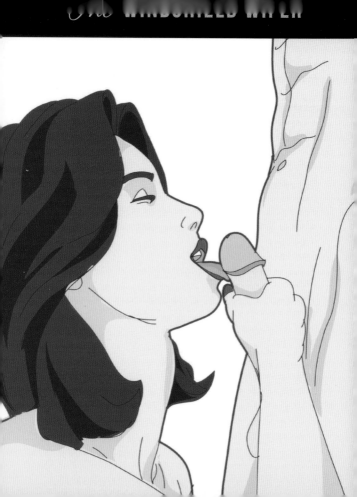

Make him crave your touch long after you're gone by exciting one of his hottest spots with your most sensual muscle: your tongue.

THE BASICS

- Use your tongue in a back and forth motion against his F-spot or frenulum. This is the hot pleasure zone on the underside of his penis where the head and shaft meet.
- Lube up your hands before wrapping them around the base of his cock so you can stroke the lower half of his shaft while performing the *Windshield Wiper*. With all that sexual stimulation, he won't know what hit him!

BLOW BY BLOW

- Have him sit up against the headboard and kneel between his bent legs.
- Wrap both hands around the base of his shaft and lower your moist lips over the head of his cock.
- Stick your tongue out against the underside of his head and slowly sweep it back and forth like windshield wipers as you suck gently with your lips.
- Try to feel his F-spot and the swollen ridge of his head with your tongue; Rotate your head ever so slightly to smooth out the sweeping motions.

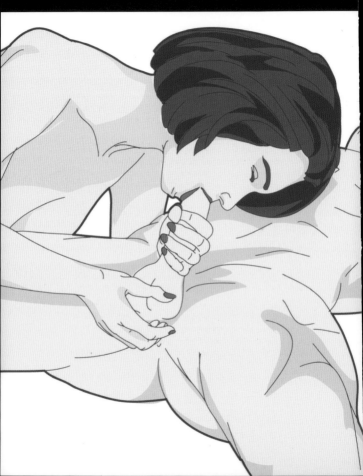

This is a move he'll never forget! Stroking and sucking from base to tip is a no-brainer for any good lover, but if you really want to take him over the edge, you'll want to extend that pleasure to his inner penis.

THE BASICS

- Seal your wet lips around his penis and suck away while your warm, wet fingers stroke the bulb of his penis through his perineum (the space between his butt and his balls).

- Since this technique requires a bit of coordination, practice in the air or on a dildo ahead of time, so that the coordinated motion of your lips and hands becomes fluid and natural.

BLOW BY BLOW

- Kneel between his legs as he sits spread eagle in an armchair.

- Wrap your lips around his cock and suck up and down from base to tip at a medium, rhythmic pace.

- As you lower your lips downward, simultaneously press your warm, lubed fingers against his perineum and stroke backward toward his butt hole.

- Imagine that your fingers are an extension of your mouth and his perineum is an extension of his penis. Stroke and suck in rhythm so that your hands move down (toward his butt) as your lips move down toward his base and your hands move up toward his balls as you suck toward the tip of his cock.

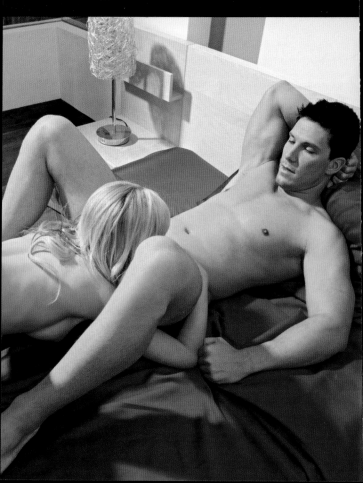

Your tongue is one of the strongest muscles in your body! But fantastic fellatio shouldn't be a workout. *The Heavyweight* leverages the weight of your body for maximum effect to leave him in awe of your sexual prowess.

THE BASICS

- Use the weight of your body to press your tongue against his shaft as you excite the sensitive underside of his penis.
- To up the ante and give him a taste of what's to come, tease him a little by adding some brief lip suction over the head of his penis when you reach the top.

BLOW BY BLOW

- Kneel between his legs as he lies flat on his back.
- Press his cock up against his abs so that the sensitive underside is revealed.
- Flatten your tongue against the base of his penis and allow the weight of your head to fall into your tongue as you press down with wet heavy pressure.
- Slide your flat tongue all the way up to the tip of his penis maintaining heavy pressure and exhaling warm air over his sensitive skin.
- As you slide back down from tip-to-base, maintain firm pressure as your tongue naturally curls around the contours of his shaft.
- Don't think of *The Heavyweight* as a *licking* move—your tongue doesn't move on its own for this technique. Instead, it moves as an extension of your head, which slides up and down and allows your tongue to stay passionately glued to his hard cock the whole time.

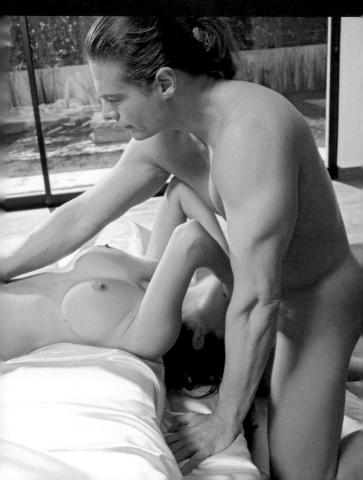

Do you both love deep throating? Well it's time to take it to the next level with a creative position that lengthens your throat and allows you to suck and swallow with serious intensity.

THE BASICS

Suck his whole cock into your mouth and use swallowing sensations to tighten your grip and pulse around the swollen base.

BLOW BY BLOW

- Lie on your back with your head hanging off the side of the bed to elongate your mouth and throat. He can slide his flavored penis into your mouth as he remains standing bedside.

- Place your hands against his hips to control the depth of penetration.

- Suck him into your mouth and gradually increase the depth as you become more relaxed.

- Once your mouth reaches the base of his penis (or your desired depth), wrap your lips around him and swallow deeply three times.

- Alternate between sucking from base to tip, performing three juicy swallows in between each sucking stroke.

- Exaggerate your swallows to create greater suction and enjoy the natural sounds of sex!

- If you find yourself gagging a little as you deep throat, you have several options:

  - If you don't mind gagging, relax and enjoy it. Don't be self-conscious, as many men (and women) are turned on by gagging sounds.

  - If gagging doesn't feel good, simply adjust your depth, and use lubed-up hands to reach deeper toward the base of his cock.

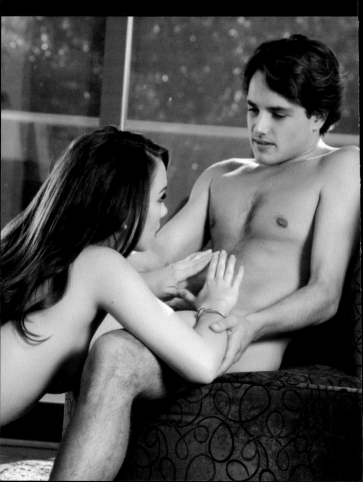

The FRENCH DO IT BETTER

Parisienne women exude this *je ne sais quoi* sex appeal, and they claim that their secret is between their legs: It's all in their panties. Even if no one will see them, it is rumored that the most beautiful French ladies always wear sexy lingerie under their clothing. To get yourself in the mood, be inspired by the French and put on some racy panties and lipstick in a color to match!

THE BASICS

Use your wet hands to form an Eiffel Tower shape over his hard cock as you gently suck his balls into your puckered lips.

BLOW BY BLOW

- Let him sit in his favorite armchair as you kneel between his legs looking up at him seductively.

- Press your moist lips into his cock as you kiss it from top to bottom working your way down to his balls, leaving bright lipstick stains over his shaft.

- Suck one of his balls into your mouth and place your lubed-up hands on either side of his shaft to create a tight seal between your palms.

- Slide your palms upward to form an Eiffel Tower over his bulging head, working up and down at a rhythmic pace.

- Learn a few French words to seduce him with. Refer to him as *mon amour* (my love), or simply respond to him with *Oui* or *Non* to set the tone.

- Be sure to slather your hands in lube for this move so that your Eiffel Tower slides smoothly up and down his shaft. The more lube you apply, the more pressure and suction you can create around his throbbing manhood.

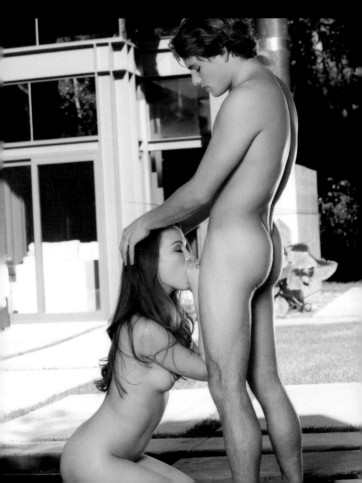

Oral sex is a matter of personal taste, and no two penises are the same. Thank goodness for variety! But since every man is different, sometimes it's best to let him take control and show you how he likes it. *Mouth Screw* requires a good degree of trust and communication as he teaches you to manhandle (or mouth-handle) his manhood to take his pleasure to new heights.

THE BASICS

Hand over the reins of control and let him penetrate your mouth however he likes it. The pleasure is all his as he adjusts the speed, depth, and intensity according to his liking.

BLOW BY BLOW

- Tell him you're craving his cock in your mouth and that you want to fulfill his every fantasy.

- Kneel at his feet as he stands bedside.

- Lick your lips and place your hands against his hips so that you can signal him with three hard taps (or the signal of your choice) if the penetration or depth gets to be too much.

- Relax and breathe slowly as he slides his hard cock in your mouth and tells you exactly what to do with your lips and tongue.

- When you need a break, offer two lubed-up hands in place of your mouth.

- The key to a great blow job is mutual enjoyment. To enjoy having a large object in your mouth, you need to be both relaxed and turned on. Before you get started with the *Mouth Screw*, kiss, rub, hump, hold his head between your legs and do whatever it takes to relax and titillate your body and mind.

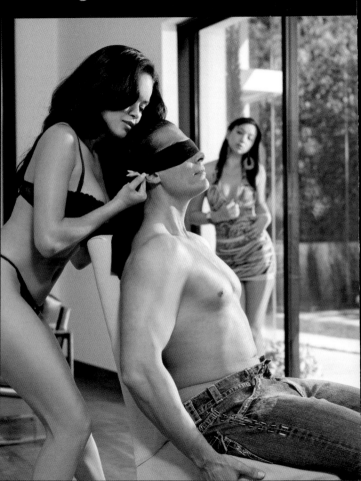

What man hasn't fantasized about having a threesome with two sexy ladies? Although neither of you may want to *live it out in reality,* playing with the *idea* of having a threesome in fantasy can be hot, hot, hot!

THE BASICS

Use a blindfold, lube, several wet body parts, and a little dirty talk to take this naughty fantasy to the next level.

BLOW BY BLOW

- Blindfold your lover so that he can focus all of his attention on your touch and your sensual whispers.

- Soak your index and middle finger in lube and "lick" one of his earlobes with your fingers while you kiss the other earlobe with your lips and tongue. The idea is to simulate two tongues at once.

- Whisper in his ear, "Do you like that? Two of us working on you at once? We want you so bad!"

- Work your two "tongues" down to his cock and "lick" up and down with both your tongue and your wet fingers so it feels like he's being serviced by two eager women.

- As you suck on his cock, use two hands to touch his balls, butt, lips, ears, perineum and shaft with your wet hands. He won't know what hit him!

- Talk dirty to him throughout the entire experience. Stroke his ego a little, reminding him how badly women crave him. Tell him that you'd love to share him and show those other girls how lucky you really are!

- Debrief after this fantasy-play and make sure you both get the reassurance you need to understand that fantasy does not have to turn into reality.

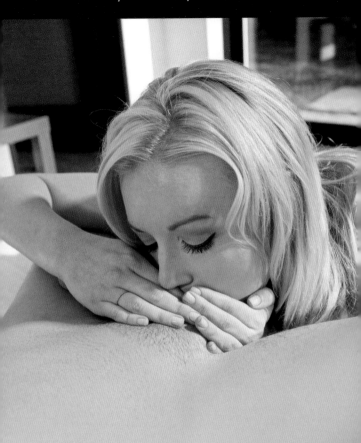

If you like blow jobs that are wet, deep, and tight, then you'll want to master the *Wet, Warm, and Wow!* By blending your hands and mouth into one seamless unit, he'll feel like he's being swallowed into a warm, moist suction tunnel that he just can't get enough of.

THE BASICS

- Use your warm, wet hands as an extension of your mouth to suck and stroke his penis from the very base to the highly sensitive tip.

- Because your hands will be the first contact point with his penis, breathe heavily as you lower your suction tunnel over his head. This will help "trick" his penis into feeling as though your hands really are a part of your extra-long mouth.

BLOW BY BLOW

- Lube up your hands and place them in prayer position in front of your face

- Press your thumbs against your lips so that your hands become an extension of your mouth. Your palms should be wet and warm, so that they feel just like your mouth.

- Lower your hands and mouth over his head, leading with your pinky fingers and squeezing as you slide down with both your hands and lips.

- Work him over at a rhythmic pace from tip to base until you can feel his cock throbbing with orgasmic release.

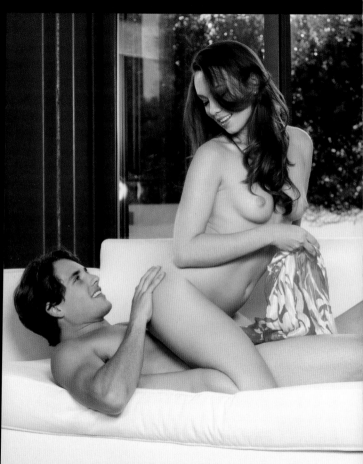

Novelty is the key to hot sex, and when you change things up, the mind and body become aroused as they anticipate something new and exciting. The simple addition of a silk scarf to the basic blow job can work wonders to heighten sensation and amplify orgasms.

THE BASICS

Suck away with your eager lips and tongue while simultaneously massaging his balls with a silk scarf.

BLOW BY BLOW

- Have you partner lie on his back and straddle his nipples so that he gets a view of your round backside.

- Lean over and suck his cock into your mouth while using both hands to drape a silk (or satin) scarf around his balls.

- Tug back and forth on the scarf with firm pressure to cup and stroke his balls as you lick, suck, and swallow his cock like a tasty popsicle.

- When he's about to finish, wrap the scarf around the base of his shaft and hold his head between your lips.

- If you're willing to sacrifice your scarf (anything for great sex, right?), lube up his balls to intensify the silky smooth sensation.

- If you feel self-conscious sitting with your butt in his face, blindfold him before getting started. The more relaxed you are, the more erotic it will feel for you both.

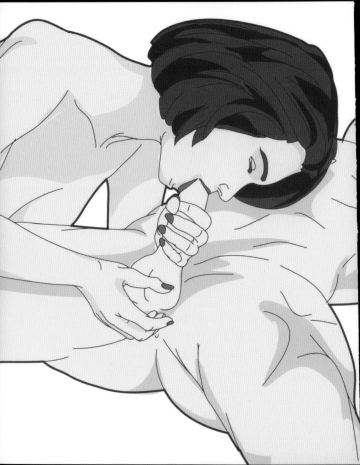

Send his body into sensation overload by pleasuring all of his hot zones at once. From the inner bulb of his penis to the very tip of his cock, using your hands, lips, and tongue to activate the genital sensory cortex of his brain will allow the orgasmic response to spread to the rest of his body.

THE BASICS

- Use you lips and tongue to pleasure his head while one hand strokes his shaft and the other takes care of his scrotum and perineum (the skin between his balls and his butt).

- Alternate hands between his shaft and perineum to change up the sensations (for him) and avoid hand cramps (for you).

BLOW BY BLOW

- Start by tracing a figure-eight over his perineum with three wet fingers. Work your way up to his balls and cup them in your wet hand, tugging down on them gently.

- Use your other hand to stroke the shaft of his cock with lots of lube, and add a firm squeeze or pulse each time you reach the base.

- At the same time, suck on the upper portion of his cock while twisting your tongue around his swollen corona.

- Though you want to pay attention to all of his hot spots, breathe deeply and do what comes naturally as you find a comfortable rhythm between your hands and mouth.

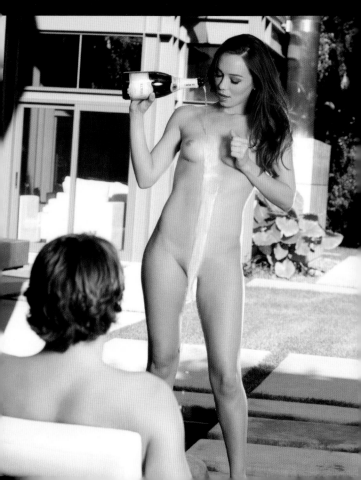

Set a celebratory tone for the evening by popping a bottle of bubbly and enjoying the tingly sensations in your mouths as you kiss. Once you take the tingly thrill south of the border, you'll have him eating out of the palm of your hand and primed to return the favor.

THE BASICS

- Take a sip of champagne (or sparkling wine) and hold a little in your mouth before drinking him in.
- Bringing food and drink into the bedroom is a simple way to spice up your sex life. Because both food/drink and sex activate the dopamine system of the brain (associated with pleasure and reward), they make the perfect pairing for mind-blowing sex.

BLOW BY BLOW

- Take a few sips of champagne and warm up with some deep kissing.
- Drizzle a little champagne over your breasts and ask him to lick it off of your nipples.
- Kneel down at his feet while he leans against the wall and run your wet lips over his balls. Positioning is important, because if you tilt your head forward, all the champagne will run out of your mouth.
- Get him primed by licking the head of his cock and running it over your lips as though you're applying lipstick with no precision.
- Take another sip of champagne, but don't swallow. Suck him into your mouth, allowing the bubbles to pop around his head.
- Twirl the liquid around your mouth as you suck up and down his shaft.
- Once the bubbles dissipate, swallow and take another small sip before returning to your *Champagne BJ*.

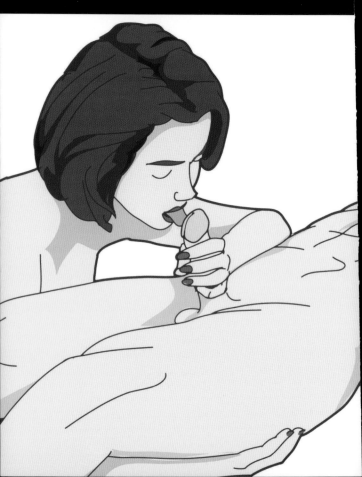

The body may be full of steamy erogenous zones, but his *million dollar point* and his *f-spot* are ones that you definitely want to pay attention to. Spoil them with love, and you'll have him eating out of the palm of your hand.

THE BASICS

You can find his *million dollar point,* otherwise known as the perineum, on the fleshy part of his skin just in front of his butt hole. This area is rich in nerve endings and is connected to the pathways that reach both his prostate (the male G-spot) and the bulb of his penis (the swollen part of the spongy tissue that surrounds his sensitive urethra). His *f-spot* is the frenulum, which is a small band of tissue located on the underside of his penis just below the head.

BLOW BY BLOW

- Lie side by side on the bed and wrap one hand around the base of his shaft.
- Suck away at a rhythmic pace until you can feel his cock throbbing with intense delight.
- As you suck toward the top of his shaft, feel his frenulum between your lips and sweep your tongue over it in a J-shape with firm pressure to make him squirm.
- Simultaneously, reach down between his legs and use all five fingers (with lube) to stroke in an oval shape over his million dollar point.
- Continue sucking, sweeping, and stroking, even as he reaches orgasm.
- If you feel his cock pulsing in your mouth, orgasm is likely imminent. Don't stop, but you may want to ease the pressure on his head and frenulum, as a lighter touch over these innervated areas is often preferable at climax.

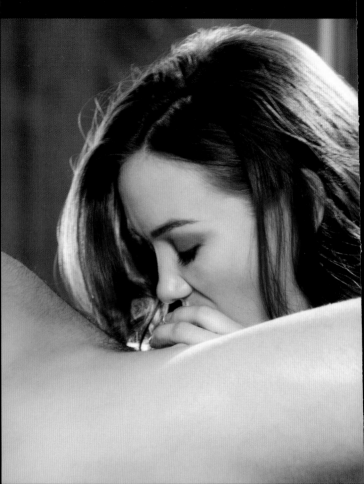

The *Catch and Release* is sure to make him moan as you use your moist lips to draw all of his sexual energy to his most sensitive region: the tip of his cock. Alternating between strong suction and a warm lip caresses will keep him guessing (and smiling) and take him to a new level of bliss beyond anything he's ever dreamed of.

THE BASICS

Use lots of suction to work your way up his shaft toward the tip and then switch it up and tease him a little as you release your lips on your way back down.

BLOW BY BLOW

- Moisten your lips and lower them down his shaft as far as you can go.

- Seal your wet lips around him as you suck upward toward the tip with all of your power and passion. Imagine that you're sucking all of his cum and sexual energy into your mouth.

- When you reach the tip, release your grip and keep your lips resting softly against his head.

- Lower your moist lips back down his shaft while breathing out gently *without* suction or firm pressure.

- Keep working up and down his shaft with firm suction on the way up and gentle cradling on the way down.

- If you want to make him come, increase the speed and keep your suction and breathing rhythmic to finish him off.

- Lube makes blow jobs better by warming it up, keeping it slippery, and protecting his manhood from any incidental teeth contact! Use your favorite flavored lube to take your pleasure and his orgasm to new heights.

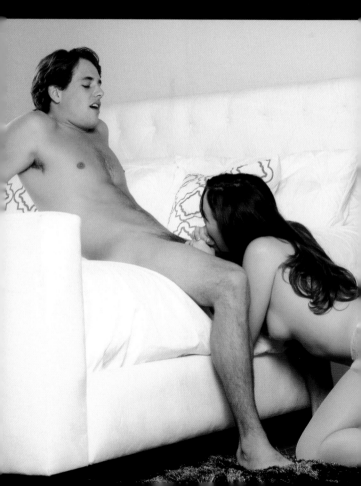

Sucking, licking, and stroking are hot, but there is something even more intense about having your most prized asset surrounded by a firm, wet tongue. The *Tongue 'n' Groove* works wonders on his cock, as the suction of your tongue can cover a considerably larger surface than your lips.

THE BASICS

- Wrap your tongue around the underside of his cock and suck away!

- Practice this move on your middle finger to get a feel for the cradling and sucking sensation with your tongue. You can start by rolling your tongue into a tube to warm up your muscles.

BLOW BY BLOW

- Kneel on the floor next to the bed as your lover lies on his back with his legs hanging off and feet flat on the floor.

- Wrap both hands around the bottom third of his cock, interlacing your fingers to create a firm seal.

- Suck the top two-thirds into your mouth, and press your tongue into the underside of his cock as hard as you possibly can. Allow it to wrap around and form a cradle squeezing the sides and bottom as you suck and slurp feverishly.

- Try to create suction with your tongue as opposed to your lips, which simply wrap around him for warmth and slippery moisture.

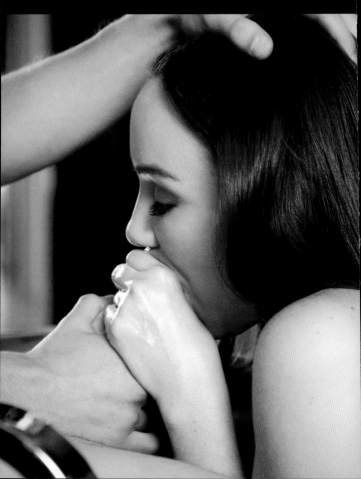

This is the perfect finishing move for the man who gets off on being in control. And with him in the driver's seat, you'll perfect your technique and reap your own climactic rewards.

THE BASICS
Let his hands guide you as you run your tongue over one of his most tender erogenous zones and you stroke yourselves into an orgasmic trance.

BLOW BY BLOW
- Kneel at his feet (he can sit on a chair or stand against the wall) and tell him that you'll do whatever you're told.

- Slather your hands in lube and wrap both of them around his shaft with your fingers interlaced. Ask him to show you how he likes it and guide your hands to find the perfect stroke, pressure, and pace.

- Once you've found the ideal rhythm, tuck your head behind his balls and press your tongue into his perineum, making large sweeping strokes in tempo with your hands.

- He may set the pace for *The Boss*, but this technique puts you in synch with one another, so it's the perfect opportunity to unite your orgasms. Strap on or insert your favorite vibrating toy or wrap yourself around his legs and grind to your heart's content.

- Play up your submissive role with a little dirty talk:

    - "Show me how to do it. You're my man."

    - "If I'm good, will you let me suck it?"

    - "I need two hands for your huge cock."

    - "I'll do anything to taste your hot cum!"

    - "I'm only here to please you."

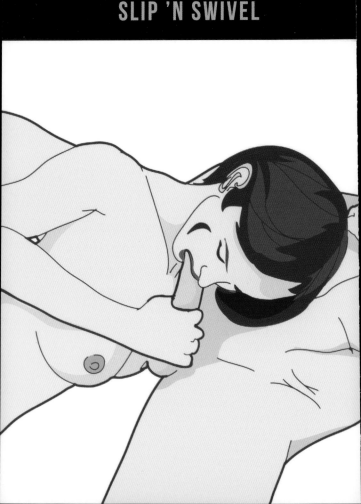

Do you ever wonder what the pros do differently to keep men lined up on their doorsteps? Aside from no-strings attached sex, they have a few tricks up their sleeve, and the *Slip 'n' Swivel* is one of their hottest pro secrets. It makes him tingle from base to tip, and by paying extra attention to his corona (that swollen ridge at the base of his head), it's sure to produce an out-of-this-world orgasmic reaction.

THE BASICS
Suck with all your might from base to tip, and twist passionately around his corona using your lips and tongue to trace its curves.

BLOW BY BLOW
- Get him all riled up with some tongue play: lick all around his balls, up and down his shaft, and press your tongue against his meatus (pee hole) while grasping his base with two warm hands.

- When you're ready to finish him off, lower your lips all the way to the base (or as deep as you feel comfortable going) and press the roof of your mouth firmly into his rock hard cock.

- Suck upward, and when you're two-thirds of the way up, swivel your head to the right and let your tongue wrap around his corona. As you slip and swivel around his cock, maintain constant suction.

- Allow your sucking, slipping, swiveling, and flicking to become one smooth movement as you lower back down to the base.

- Repeat until you feel the waves of orgasmic pleasure pulsating through his penis.

- Let your slurps, sucks, and other natural sex sounds run wild! Sex is supposed to be a sensual experience, and sound is an often-under-valued erotic sense. So don't hold back. Breathe deeply and let your naughty noises come out to play!

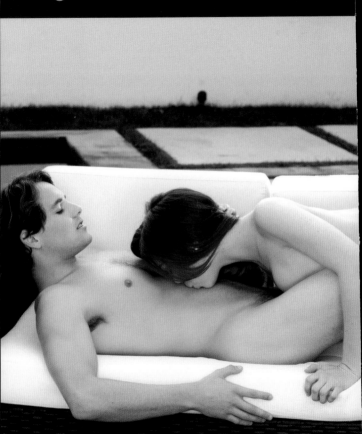

Suction, lubrication, and rhythm are elemental to any good blow job and *The Ultimate Indulgence* combines all three to take him over the edge.

THE BASICS

- Alternate between three deep sucks and three shallow ones to tantalize the supersensitive head, as well as the highly reactive lower third of his cock.

- Tweaking your oral movements and strokes in small ways can produce massive results, as his body and mind get excited by the unknown. By trying *The Ultimate Indulgence* in different positions (between his legs, straddling him from the top, or approaching from the side), it will feel like a whole new move each and every time as his penis comes into different points of contact with your lips and tongue.

BLOW BY BLOW

- Begin by kissing a few of his often ignored erogenous zones with loose, soft lips: try his forehead, collarbone, hipbones and that sensitive patch above his nipples.

- Once you've worked your way down, press your lips into his shaft and run them up and down, like you're eating corn on the cob but with no teeth.

- When you're both feeling relaxed and aroused, open your mouth around his head and suck four to five times with your lips wrapped around his corona (the swollen ridge).

- Lower your lips to the base, squeeze tightly, and suck four to five times at the deepest point possible, swallowing with every suck.

- Alternate between sucking on his head and base at a steady pace until you feel a pulsing sensation rushing through his shaft. At this point, take him into your mouth as deep as possible, and press your hand into his perineum (the space between his balls and butt).

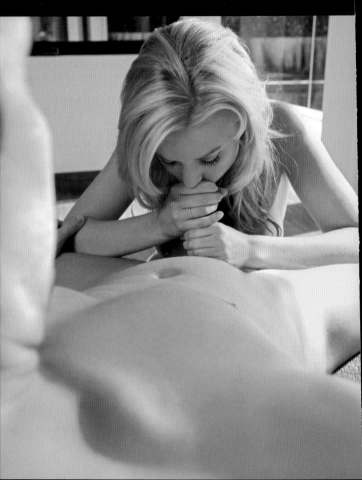

Supermodels may not have much to teach us about sex, but their over-the-top pouts do double-duty on and off-camera. Copy their classic pout to create new sensations while sucking away, and be sure to switch up your positioning using the *Supermodel* to keep him guessing and coming back for more.

THE BASICS

Blow him away using your soft, warm cheeks instead of your lips and tongue. By approaching from the side, you'll put extra pressure on the highly responsive frenulum and the sensitive dorsal vein.

BLOW BY BLOW

• Kneel at your lover's side as he lies flat on the bed and gets the perfect profile view of your curves.

• Press your tongue flat against the bottom of your mouth to cover your bottom teeth and lower your lips over his head as far as the coronal ridge.

• Suck your cheeks in like a supermodel posing for a photo and allow them to press up against his cock as you suck away.

• Overplay the sucking in sensation with your cheeks as you allow them to envelop his cock from top to bottom.

• When you need a breather, exaggerate a big swallow at the tip of his cock and allow your lips to create a popping sound as they disengage. Look up into his eyes and hold his manhood in one hand like an old fashioned video game joystick before returning to work.

• If your facial muscles get tired (the supermodel pout takes work!), press your hands against your cheeks to tighten your grip around his cock.

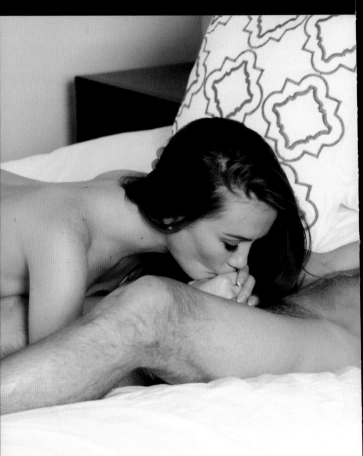

The warmth and intimacy of your mouth may be unparalleled when it comes to enveloping his cock, but add your steamy hands to the mix, and he won't know what hit him. *The Goddess* uses your hands to elongate your hot mouth and launch his body into a torrent of fervid pleasure.

THE BASICS

Create a tight suction around his shaft with your hands and attach them to your mouth as you "deep throat" his big, hard cock. If you warm them up and use enough lube, it will feel like the deepest, tightest blow job ever.

BLOW BY BLOW

- Blindfold your lover and have him lie on the bed with his legs hanging off the sides. Kneel at his feet and keep a bottle of lube handy.

- Create a suction tunnel with your hands:

  - Start in prayer position. Rotate the fingers of your right hand toward you while the fingers of your left hand slide slightly away.

  - Create a tight hole between your thumbs and another hole opposite them to form a tunnel.

- Apply lots of lube, and place your "tunnel" against your lips to create a long suction path from your pinky fingers to your throat.

- Lower your hands and lips down toward his head and exhale deeply so that he feels your breath on his head before your hands touch down.

- Suck from base to tip squeezing tightly with your palms and lips. You can use lots of pressure as long as he's lubed up.

- To finish him off, speed up your sucking to two strokes (one up and one down) per second.

- To send him into orgasmic overdrive, squeeze the base of his cock with your fingers on every stroke. This pulsing sensation mimics the orgasmic contractions he experiences when he comes.

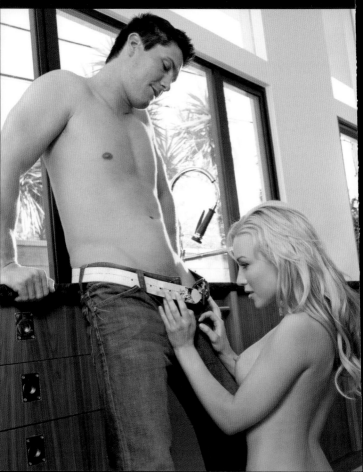

Your classic up-and-down sucking and stroking can work wonders on his throbbing member, but by changing things up, you'll keep him guessing and make him feel like it's his first time experiencing your warm, wet mouth. Light candles or lower the lights to set the mood and ensure that you feel comfortable walking around (or kneeling) naked in heels.

THE BASICS

- Suck on his cock while nodding your head in "yes" and "no" motions.
- Take *Yes! Yes! Yes!* to the next level by trying it out (on the kitchen table) in the sixty-nine position!

BLOW BY BLOW

- Greet him in the kitchen wearing nothing but stilettos and a long strand of beads around your neck.
- Ask him to sit on the counter or kitchen table, and slide yourself between his legs. Depending on the height, you can place a cushion below your knees or stand up.
- Use your hands to drip tasty lube over his cock, and gently caress his thighs with your lubed-up hands.
- Once you're both worked up, lower your lips over his lubed cock and nod your head up and down as if you're saying "Yes! Yes! Yes!"
- Perform your "yes" movements over his head and then lower halfway down his shaft and repeat.
- When you come back up to his head, press your tongue flat against him and alternate between "yes" and "no."
- Add a few full head circles, allowing your tongue to wrap all the way around his corona (the swollen ridge at the base of his head) and finish him off by stroking the lower half of his cock with a warm, wet hand while simultaneously nodding your head over the upper half with quick rhythmic movements.

COME TOGETHER!

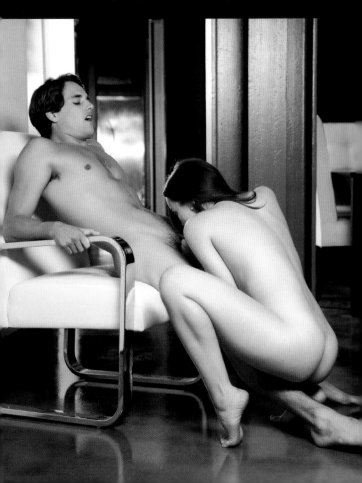

Going down doesn't have to be one-sided. If you feel a tingling while ravishing his rod, reach down and take care of yourself too!

THE BASICS

- Rub off against his calves while you give him a blow job. Control your arousal and wait for his impending orgasm before letting your orgasm flow simultaneously.

- Simultaneous orgasms can and do happen, but you don't want them to turn into a high-pressure goal. One way to learn to control your orgasm is to masturbate and practice alternating between different levels of arousal (through peaks and plateaus) before coming.

BLOW BY BLOW

- Kneel between his legs while he relaxes in an armchair. Look him in his eyes and unhook your bra, allowing the cups to rest against your breasts. Lick all around his shaft as though your tongue is dancing on a pole for his visual pleasure.

- Once he is hard, allow your bra to fall to the floor, and press your breasts around his cock as you suck teasingly on the tip. Gradually suck him deeper into your mouth with loose lips and light suction.

- By now, he should be aching for more, so wrap your lips tightly around his shaft at the deepest point you can reach and suck as hard as you can. Keep sucking as you ride his legs and rub yourself into a frenzied state of arousal.

- Time your frottage (dry humping) with your cock sucking, and wait for his cock to start pulsing intensely—this marks the point of no return and is a sure-fire indicator that he's about to come!

- Do whatever it takes to get yourself off, too—reach down with your hands, grab hold of your favorite vibrator, or fantasize about a hot sex scene so that you feel the orgasmic contractions as he comes or shortly thereafter.

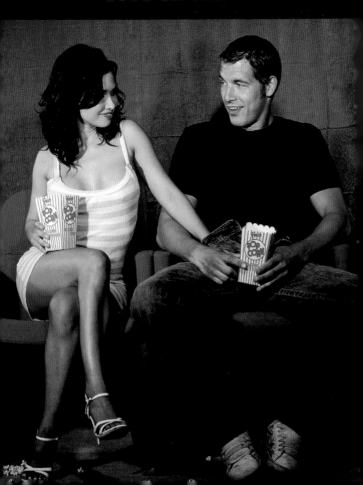

Try *Love on the Run* in a car, elevator, bus, plane, or train and enjoy the passionate aftermath that results from the thrill of public sex.

THE BASICS

- Use your hottest hands and mouth techniques to offer him a quickie on the road!

- If you want to make him come faster, alternate between tight sucking (or stroking) of the lower third of his shaft and more rapid sucking on his head. Add a twist over his corona and a ton of genuine enthusiasm, and he'll be melting in the palm of your hand in no time!

BLOW BY BLOW

- Pack the essential supplies (lube and a scarf or blanket for privacy) and choose the midpoint of your travel to initiate *Love on the Run*.

- If he's driving, turn up the music to set the mood, and if you're in a more public place (train, plane, bus, etc.), cover his lap with a scarf before unbuttoning his pants. Be sure to book the back row in advance if you have the option to do so.

- Smear lube on your hand and slather your palm all over his head and shaft. Roll your fingers around playfully without grabbing him as he starts to get hard.

- Use your other hand to touch yourself if it helps to get you in the mood.

- Twirl your tongue (or two wet fingers) around his shaft and breathe over his head. Suck his head into your mouth or wrap two wet hands around his shaft as you begin stroking. Pepper your moves with lots of "Mmm's" and "Ahhh's."

- If you like to swallow, take him deep into your throat as he comes. If you prefer to use your hands, wrap them around his coronal ridge during orgasm and use your scarf to manage the sexy mess.

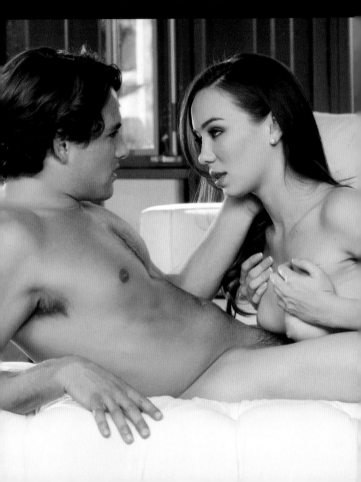

There is more to a facial than simply coming on a lover's face. Oral sex is a highly personal act, and its intimacy can be intensified with some passionate eye contact, naughty-but-nice dirty talk, and erotic voyeurism.

THE BASICS

Rub your face all over his cock and balls and encourage him to relish in the thrill of watching himself come all over your breasts, stomach, mouth, or face.

BLOW BY BLOW

- Position yourself so he has a nice view of your face between his legs.

- Draw his head into your mouth and press it into your cheeks so that he can see its shape through your cheeks. Close your lips to pop him out and run the tip of his cock over your lips while looking up into his eyes.

- Lick him with a slobbery tongue from base to tip, and rub his shaft up and down the side of your face. Offer a genuine compliment, such as "I love your cock!" "It's so big in my mouth!" or "I just want to taste you!"

- Suck him into your mouth and take breaks to rub him all over your cheeks, lips, and chin. When he's ready to come, tell him you want to watch, and feel his hot load against your skin.

- Grab him by the base and point it wherever you want it: in your open mouth, all over your breasts, on your stomach, or on your face.

- Coming on a lover's face is a top fantasy for many men. Some claim that it's an act of degradation (which can be a part of consensual power play), while others suggest that it's more about acceptance and validation because it's so common in mainstream porn. No consensual act is inherently degrading; nor is any sex act inherently empowering. Sex, pleasure, and power are yours to negotiate, and only you can define what gets you off.

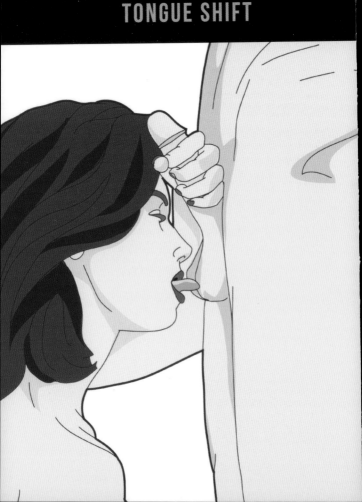

The nerve-rich head of his cock is not only sensitive to your touch, but also to temperature, texture, and moisture. Shift your tongue's positioning and movements to play with variety and spark new sensations in this highly erogenous area.

THE BASICS

- Suck on his throbbing head while alternating between your upper and lower tongue to provide extra stimulation to his frenulum (the little notch on the underside of the penis just below the head).

- Modify the *Tongue Shift* by using the topside of your tongue to stroke his frenulum and then stimulating the upper side of his head with the underside of your tongue. It sounds complicated, but if you try it on your finger first, it will flow smoothly.

BLOW BY BLOW

- Resist the urge to suck him into your mouth right away. Instead, flutter your tongue along his abdomen and around the base of his shaft.

- Run your tongue along his raphe (the dividing line that stretches from his anus over the center of his perineum and balls up to the tip of his cock) and blow cool air over your wet path.

- Suck him into your mouth and alternate between twirling your lips around his head and pressing your tongue into his lower shaft while maintaining suction.

- As he becomes more aroused, focus on his frenulum and flatten the top of your tongue against it while sucking. Switch it up and continue sucking while pressing the ridged underside of your tongue against this sweet spot. You'll need to bend your tongue backwards to execute this move.

- Keep the suction and wetness constant while shifting between the topside and underside of your tongue every ten seconds.

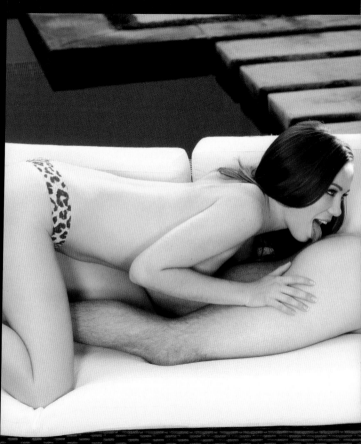

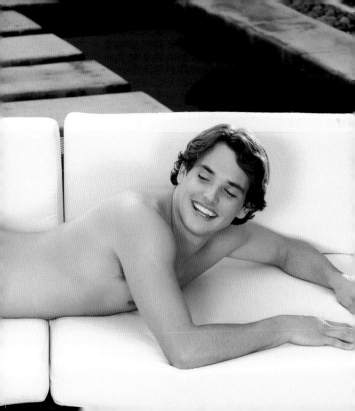

Anal play and rimming (licking, sucking, and kissing the anus) can lead to overpowering sexual response and orgasms for both men and women. The anus is packed with responsive nerve endings, and many couples consider the backside indispensable to their steamy oral sex repertoire.

THE BASICS

- Ease into rimming gradually by working your way around your lover's delicate pucker before diving in for some hot and heavy sucking, kissing, and caressing.

- Communication is of paramount importance to any sexual experience—especially if you're trying something new. Whether you happen to be the giver or the taker, be sure to ask for and offer lots of constructive feedback.

PLAY BY PLAY

- The techniques below are merely guidelines. You don't have to follow each tip sequentially. If you find something that works, stick with it!

- Plant feather-light kisses with wet lips all over your lover's butt cheeks.

- Add your tongue to your kisses, wiggling it in between his butt cheeks.

- Apply your favorite flavored lube and rub it in with two thumbs.

- Press your tongue flat against the pucker (bum hole) and curl it upwards.

- Paint, twirl, and lick around your lover's pucker teasingly.
- Swivel your tongue in a figure-eight over their perineum and bum hole.
- Use two hands to spread your lover's butt cheeks and press your lips around the pucker while twirling your tongue in circular motions.
- Change directions with your tongue and widen your licks into large ovals. Alternate between wet oval-shaped strokes with a wide, flat tongue and short flicks with just the tip.
- When you're both feeling ready and relaxed, stick out your tongue and glide the tip in and out of the pucker. Your lover will need to relax to allow your soft tongue to slide in.
- Wiggle your tongue up and down, side to side, and in circular motions as you penetrate your lover's warm pucker.
- Reach one lubed-up hand around and stroke his cock in rhythm with your sucking and licking.

FOR HER

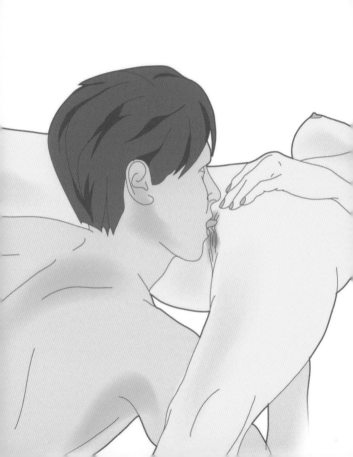

Combine the pinpoint accuracy of your tongue with the power of your fingers as you spread the erotic tingle back to the outer edges of her G-spot (the area on the upper wall of the vagina associated with gusher orgasms).

THE BASICS

- Spread your fingers over her G-spot to form a peace sign while your tongue strokes her clitoral hood.

- If she loves to squirt, add the ring finger and some pelvic pressure into the mix! Open and close all three fingers (index, middle, and ring) in a "W" formation over her swollen G-spot while pressing down on her lower abdomen with your other hand.

LICK BY LICK

- Kneel at her feet as she lies on the bed with her legs hanging off the edge.

- Press your tongue against the very top of her vulva over the hood of her clit and the bottom of her Venus mound. Lick up and down with short strokes, alternating between the top and the underside of your tongue to vary the texture and sensations.

- Slide your wet index and middle fingers into her pussy with your palm facing upward and press against her upper vaginal wall feeling for the swollen ridge-like area of her G-spot.

- When you're as deep as your second knuckles, spread your fingers apart to form a peace sign and close them rhythmically as though they're a pair of scissors.

- Time your tongue strokes to align with your finger movements to pleasure her clitoris and G-spot in perfect rhythm.

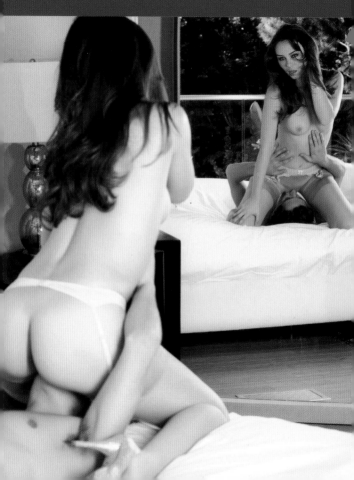

If she likes to watch, this one is right up her alley! She gets to take in the sexy view while you lie back and eat her out to your heart's content.

THE BASICS

- Position a mirror in front of your bed so that she can watch you writhe in pleasure between her legs.
- Press your hands into her butt cheeks to pull her pussy into your face and intensify the pressure, thrusting, and pleasure.

LICK BY LICK

- Have her kneel on the mattress facing her reflection in the mirror.
- Lie on your back with your face beneath her pussy and your feet behind her, away from the mirror. Place enough pillows under your head to support your neck while you lick, suck, kiss, and slurp away!
- Begin by teasing her inner lips (the ones that usually hang lower) with the soft tip of your nose. Breathe in and tell her you love her scent.
- Stick your tongue out as far as you can and use only the tip to trace the space between her inner and outer lips so that she can watch your tongue in the mirror.
- Pull your head forward a little (toward the mirror) and wrap your lips around as much of her as possible while sucking gently.
- As she gets more excited, reach up toward her clitoris with your tongue and pulse against her with firm pressure.
- If she gets tired or sore while kneeling, she can put her hands down and rest on all fours.

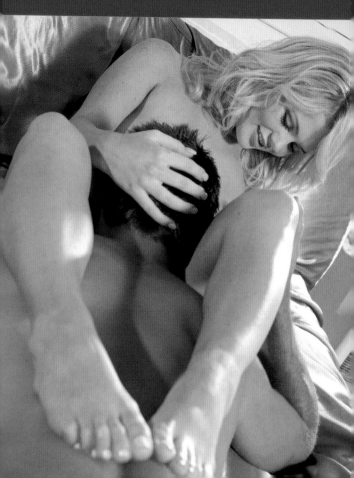

Giving is grand, but sometimes being selfish makes for the most sizzling sex! *The Remote Control* is all about her animalistic desire to take exactly what she wants. As you submit to her oral needs, the power of being in control will excite her inner dominatrix while you'll have a chance to relish in her carnal pleasure.

THE BASICS

Let her use her hands to guide your head as you eat her out with delight.

LICK BY LICK

- Look her in the eye and tell her that you want to ravish her and cater to her every need.

- As she sits on the edge of the bed with her legs dangling off the side, kneel on the floor at her feet.

- Place her hands on the back of your head and tell her you want her to show you how she likes it.

- Encourage her to control the speed, pressure, direction, and strokes by directing your head with her hands.

- Look up at her and ask her if she wants it harder, softer, slower, or faster.

- Remind her how much you love it and how badly you want to please her.

- Create a private code to communicate during oral sex. For example, two taps to the back of your head means she wants you to speed up, while a gentle tug of your ear indicates that she wants you to slow down. Play with these sexy codes in and out of the bedroom to build sexual tension throughout the week.

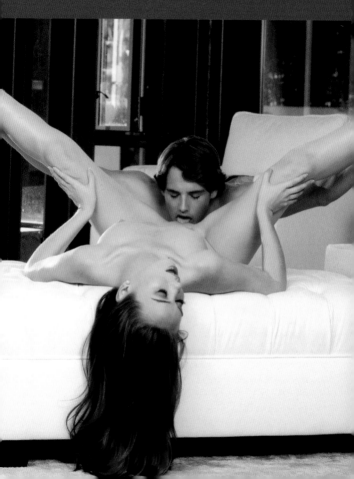

What woman hasn't fantasized about being ravaged by a real-life Casanova or Christian Grey? It may sound too good to be true, but with a little confidence and a few sure-fire moves, you can leave her begging for more and more of what you've got!

THE BASICS

- Hold her legs up in the air, drop to your knees, and make her moan with delight.

- Take deep breaths and moan as you eat her out. It will help her to relax and elicit her own natural sex sounds.

LICK BY LICK

- Look her in the eye and tell her that you've been craving her all day long.

- Kiss her on the lips and lay her on her back at the edge of the bed.

- Grab her ankles in one hand and throw her legs up in the air as you drop to your knees on the floor. Allow your hand to slide down her legs if necessary, but keep a tight grip, and promise her that you're going to make her scream.

- Press your tongue flat against her bum hole and pulse 4-5 times before licking your way to her fourchette (the sweet spot where her lower lips meet). Stop here again and pulse another 4-5 times.

- Lick your lips and press them into her pussy sliding all the way to the top and twirling your tongue around her clitoris.

- Continue licking and kissing a long line between her bum hole and her clit until she is pressing her pussy into you and begging for more.

- Once she's worked up, moan with desire as you open wide and suck her entire pussy into your mouth.

- Alternatively, you can use two hands to hold her legs in the air and spread them wide apart for easy access.

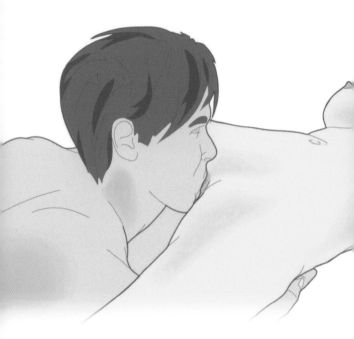

Combining the suction of your warm lips with some targeted tongue dexterity can be tricky, but it's well worth the practice. The *Tight Twirl* allows you to suck and stimulate her entire vulva, which is packed with erogenous tissue and thousands of nerve endings!

THE BASICS

- Open wide, and press your lips against her vulva while creating suction and twirling your tongue around the perimeter.

- Multitasking makes for great lovers, so keep those hands busy! Rub them against her thighs, buttocks, and breasts as you suck and twirl between her legs.

LICK BY LICK

- Choose your favorite position, and open your mouth around her pussy as wide as you can.

- Suck gently with your lips as you trace your tongue in a big oval around the inside of the tight lip seal. Your tongue stays pressed against your lips as it twirls around, and you should hear the sweet sounds of suction as your twirl in one direction.

- Alternate the direction of your tongue twirling, and pepper a few bottom-to-top licks between your sensual circles.

- As she gets more excited, you can slide your tongue into her vagina while maintaining the suction cup of your moist lips.

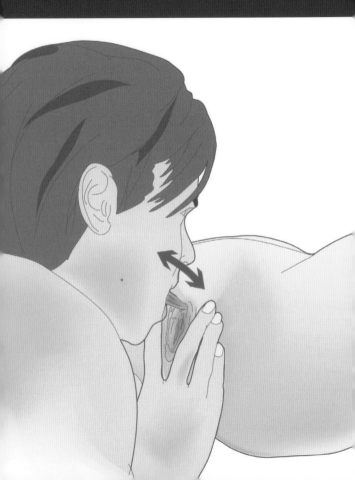

An eager lover who dives right in with passion and lust is sometimes all it takes to put her in the mood and bring her to the heights of orgasmic bliss. So, don't be shy! The *Open Sesame* offers the ideal balance between her vulnerability and your assured attentiveness to let her feel like a lady—once, twice, and three times over.

THE BASICS

- Use your fingers to pry open her juicy lips and make way for your talented tongue.

- If she's shy about opening her legs wide and letting you dive in, get her permission to tie her legs spread eagle against your bed posts (or the legs of a wide armchair) before going down on her.

LICK BY LICK

- Caress her thighs with some edible massage oil or lube to help put her in the mood.

- Look down between her legs and then look up into her eyes and tell her she's beautiful. Then, smile as you lower your head and pry open her lips with your fingers.

- Breathe gently over her opening and tell her how desperate you are to taste it.

- Rub your cheeks against her open lips before licking across the opening horizontally from side to side and then diagonally from top to bottom.

- Suck on the opening, and point the tip of your tongue into her vagina, gradually increasing the depth and allowing your face to press flat against her wet spot.

- Curl your tongue upward and feel her G-spot as the tip of your nose rests gently against her clit.

- Alternate between tongue strokes, tongue insertions, and lip sucking, paying attention to her unique responses, sounds, and movements.

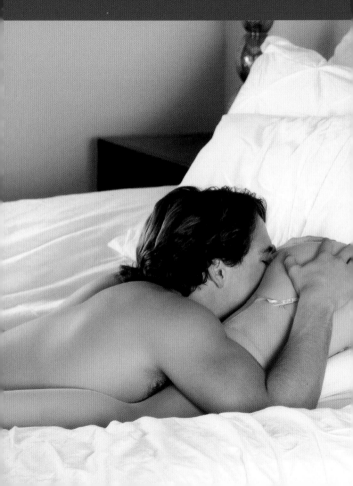

BACK DOOR DINING

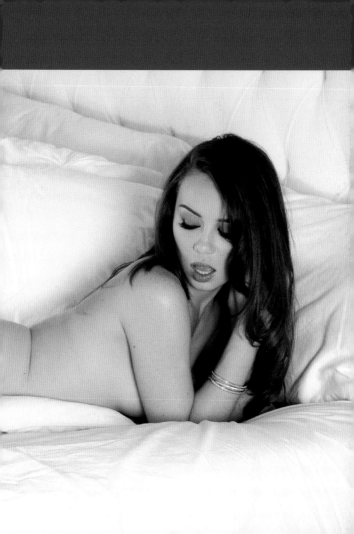

BACK DOOR DINING

Change up your positioning to give yourself a sexy view and allow her to experience your orgasm-inducing tongue tricks from a brand new angle.

THE BASICS

- Eat her out from behind and make her ache for more as you work your way up to her sensitive clitoris oh-so-slowly.

- Many women learn to orgasm while lying on their stomachs, so she may be an expert in this position. Encourage her to reach down between her legs with her hand while you eat her out so that her orgasm becomes a team effort.

LICK BY LICK

- Roll her onto her stomach and lie between her spread legs as you slide your hands under her hips. You may also want to prop them up with a few pillows on either side.

- Use a wide, flat tongue to paint slow figure-eights over her perineum (the soft patch between her labia and bum). Breathe slowly and deeply to encourage her to relax and do the same.

- After 10–12 figure-eight strokes, add a third circle to your figure eight, working your way forward toward her pussy. Keep adding extra circles until you reach her inner lips, and then curl your tongue upward to penetrate her with its firm tip.

- Work your way up to the top of her pussy so your nose and forehead are buried in her backside while your tongue circles her clitoris.

- Press your lips into her and suck away, allowing the natural wet sounds to emanate from your lips and hers.

- Encourage her to relax and allow her hips to thrust into your face while your hands help her to find the perfect rhythm.

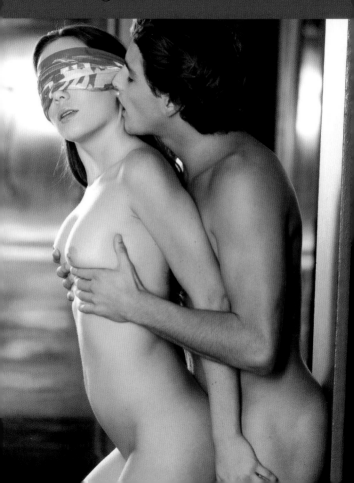

Some women can actually reach orgasm from having their breasts fondled, sucked, and kissed. Use this move to put our verified claims to the test.

THE BASICS

- Tease and stimulate the area above her nipples and beneath her warm breasts to bring her to a mind-blowing orgasm. One breast (and one nipple) is usually more sensitive than the other, so find out which side your lady favors. Erotic sensitivity on the left side is more common, but the only way to know is to ask!

- Tell her how great her tits are too! Compliments are a powerful aphrodisiac.

LICK BY LICK

- Let her lie on her side comfortably with a pillow beneath her head and knees as you lie facing her. Blindfold her to help her focus on the erotic sensations. Caress her face, neck, and collarbone as gently as possible with your fingertips.

- Don't grab or knead her breasts. Instead, use soft open palms to lightly encircle her nipples as you kiss her neck.

- The area above her nipples is often the most sensitive, so kiss, lick, and suck around this erogenous zone for a few minutes before working your way around the outer edges.

- Continue kissing and sucking around her outer curves until you arrive at the bottom of her breasts, where you can use your tongue to lick under their soft folds.

- Gradually work your way from the outer edge with sloppy wet, suction-cup kisses until you arrive at her nipples. Blow on them gently.

- Suck on her nipples with a wide, loose mouth to tease and tantalize them before closing your tight lips and flicking your tongue around in circular motions.

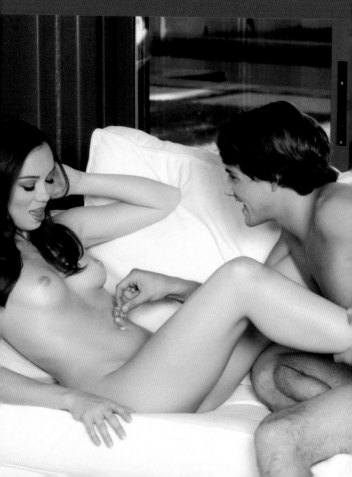

MAKE HER PURR

Vibrator orgasms rank as some of the most intense experiences for many women. Owning a vibrating toy is actually linked to higher levels of overall sexual satisfaction. So, combine your tongue's natural skill with some sweet vibrating sensations to trigger her orgasmic platform and launch her pleasure into a whole new realm.

THE BASICS

- Wrap a vibrating cock rick around the base of your tongue before you begin your expert muff-diving session.

- As an alternative to using a cock ring on your tongue, you can learn to use her favorite hand-held vibrator and create a new shared routine with your hands, fingers, and tongue.

LICK BY LICK

- Wrap a stretchy (silicone) cock ring with a built-in vibrator around the base of your tongue.

- Select the lowest setting as you begin to lick up and down her outer lips with just the tip of your tongue.

- Increase the pressure of your licks as you flatten your tongue to cover a greater area. Pretend you're licking a soft-serve ice cream cone, and don't worry about the vibrator touching her skin directly, as your tongue will pass along the vibrations.

- When her body starts to squirm with pleasure, turn up the vibrations and press the underside of your tongue into her vagina. Use your fingers to hold her lips open if needed.

- Roll your tongue around the inside wall of her vagina in a wide circular motion, allowing the vibrations to travel inside her orgasmic platform (the area on the outer third of the vaginal canal).

- Ask her to show you where she wants to be touched, and press the bullet-end of the vibrating ring firmly into this hot spot as she wanders off into a deep, unforgettable orgasm.

BEGGING FOR MORE

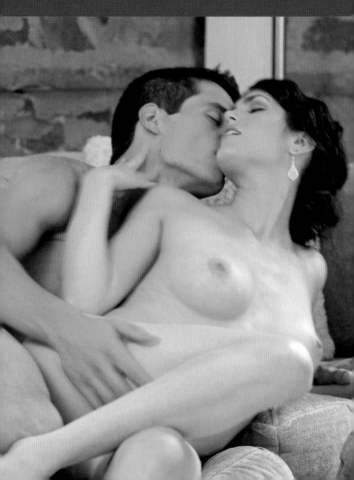

You already know how to find and fondle her hottest spots, but if you want to intensify and multiply her orgasms, sometimes you need to tease her into a desperate frenzy. It may require of bit of self-restraint on your part, but the rapturous rewards are well worth the wait.

THE BASICS

- Fondle and titillate her entire body, avoiding her hottest erogenous zones to make them palpitate with desire. When you finally give her what she's begging for, her entire body will tingle with climactic pleasure.

- When her body is overtaken by orgasmic waves of pleasure, press the top of your tongue flat against her vulva and hold it in place firmly to feel her wet orgasmic contractions.

LICK BY LICK

- Lay your lover down on her stomach and place a pillow under her hips.

- Kiss her outer ears with wet, loose lips before working your way down to the nape of her neck. Trace a line down her spine with your tongue and breathe heavily over the small of her back.

- Run your tongue between her booty cheeks and down between the slit in her thighs before slowly kissing your way down her inner legs to her ankles.

- Roll her over onto her back, and rub your face, tongue, and lips all over her thighs. Allow your face to fleetingly brush up against her aching pussy, but don't pay it any purposeful attention—yet.

- Kiss all around her breasts, but don't touch her nipples. Blow warm air over them, resisting the urge to kiss or suck.

- Kiss a trail from between her breasts to the top of her pussy and blow gentle kisses over her labia without making physical contact.

- Keep teasing by kissing, sucking, and caressing all around her hot spots until she starts thrusting her hips into you.

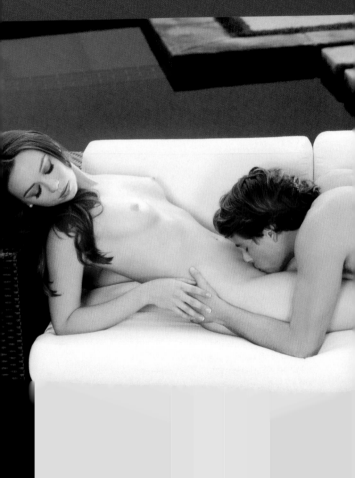

LUSTY LOINS

The way we masturbate during our early sexual years leaves a lasting imprint on our arousal and experiences of pleasure for years to come. Because so many women learn to orgasm by rubbing their legs together or wrapping them around a firm object, it's no surprise that this rubbing sensation becomes an essential component of their lifelong orgasms. Take advantage of this go-to self-pleasure secret to "screw" her thighs while simultaneously stimulating her sensitive *mons*, clitoris and labia.

THE BASICS

Squeeze her thighs together to create tight friction and use your hands, toys, and cock to rub her into a state of orgasmic bliss.

LICK BY LICK

- Start with some simple tongue screwing: use your tongue like a small penis to penetrate her, sliding in and out of her vagina as deep as you can reach. Don't be afraid to let your face (nose, cheeks, and forehead) press flat against her vulva.

- Just as her body begins to beg for more of your slick tongue, grab hold of her outer thighs and squeeze her legs together. Slide your tongue into the crease of her inner thighs and twirl it around the warm, wet space.

- Continue to "screw" her thighs with your tongue, hand (with lube), cock, or favorite vibrating toy. As you glide in and out, be sure to press upward against her vulva.

- Tell her to squeeze her thighs together to heighten the friction and use her hips to guide the pace.

- Some women can reach orgasm simply from rubbing their thighs together or crossing their legs. These movements can stimulate the clitoral nerves and activate the muscles of her pelvic floor that contract during orgasm.

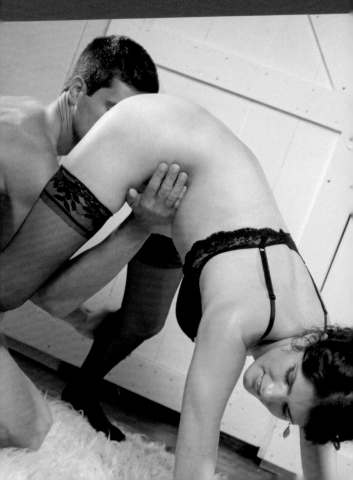

Playing with the butt may be taboo, but that's part of what makes it so erotic and exciting. Combine the thrill of the forbidden with all those sensual nerve endings and you've got the perfect recipe for out-of-this-world orgasms.

THE BASICS

- Suck on and kiss her pucker (bum hole) while you use your fingers to fondle her sensitive perineum.

- If you want to combine the *Bootylicious* with some good old fashioned pussy-eating, be sure to remember the pussy-first rule: you can move from her pussy to her anus, but not the other way around, as you don't want to transfer bacteria from the bum to the vagina.

LICK BY LICK

- If it's your first time approaching her back door, talk to her first to make sure she's ready. Sex talk doesn't have to be clinical. You can begin with, "I love your ass. I just want to run my tongue between your hot cheeks. Would you like that?"

- Have her lie on her stomach with a pillow propping up her hips.

- Kiss the upper part of her butt cheeks and the small of her back with wide puckered lips as you trace circles toward the mid-line of her bum.

- Pull her butt cheeks apart with your hands as you slide the tip of your tongue down toward her hole.

- Flatten your tongue against her and twirl it around in a circular motion. Try painting flower petals around her pucker.

- If she likes it, slide your pointy tongue inside and continue to twirl it around.

- Release her butt cheeks from your hands and continue to thrust your tongue in and out of her as you reach under with one hand to pet her perineum with soft, whispery finger strokes.

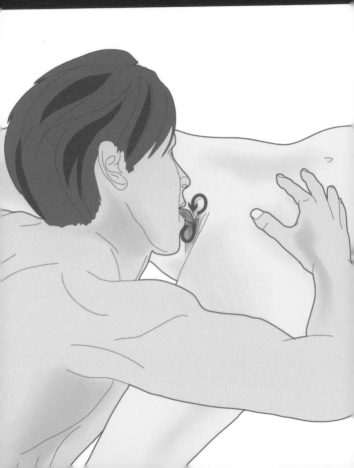

By mimicking the sensation of orgasmic contractions, this technique not only produces powerful orgasms, but also can prolong the climactic euphoria and promote multiples.

THE BASICS

- Pulse over her hot spots with your tongue and/or fingers as she approaches orgasm.

LICK BY LICK

- Before trying this super-steamy finishing move, find out where your lover likes to be touched during orgasm. You can watch her finish herself off or simply ask her for a little guidance.

- Lick all around the outer edges of her vulva as you slide your middle finger in and out of her wet pussy. Alternate screwing her with your tongue and fingers, licking up any wetness that drips down her legs.

- As her hips undulate with greater speed and intensity, it is likely a sign that climax is imminent, and it's time to bring on the *Sexual Heartbeat*. Tailor this move to her specific hot spots by pressing and releasing every half-second. You have several options including:

    - Cupping your entire hand around her vulva like a Jill-strap.

    - Pressing the underside of your tongue against her clitoris.

    - Curling your index and middle fingers inside of her and press up into her G-spot on the upper vaginal wall.

    - Using your tongue or fingers to press against her pucker as she moans and writhes with pleasure.

- As she comes, keep your pulsing consistent even as the speed and intensity of her contractions subside to promote longer, multiple experiences of orgasmic pleasure.

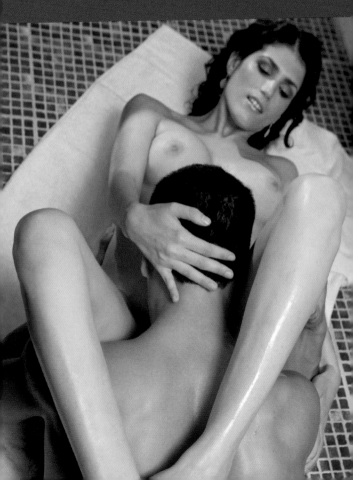

Female ejaculation (squirting) has likely been around since the dawn of time, and those who experience it often relish in the wet and wild rapture. And though it's not a sideshow trick, if your lady likes to indulge in a little G-spot action, she may just go equally gaga for a gusher orgasm.

THE BASICS

Titillate her G-spot from both sides to bring her over the edge and encourage her to release a torrent of orgasmic energy. Try the *Sultry Squirter* in the shower or lay a few towels down to avoid any concerns of creating a mess.

LICK BY LICK

• Kiss, fondle, and caress her body to heighten her arousal. When she's ready, insert your middle and ring finger into her vagina pulling up against the upper wall.

• Alternate between a come hither motion over her G-spot and a tick-tock movement from side to side with both fingers. You will likely feel her G-spot swell as you fondle it.

• Suck rhythmically on her clitoris with your lips as you continue stroking her G-spot with two fingers.

• As she becomes more aroused, place your other hand flat on her mons (the flesh over the pubic bone) and lower abdomen and undulate it in unison with your come hither strokes. This will allow you to stimulate her urethral sponge (the site of the G-spot) from both the abdominal/bladder wall and the vaginal interior. Encourage her to breathe deeply and bear down as she is overtaken by orgasm.

• The experience of squirting varies from person to person. Some dribble a few drops while others spray with considerable force, but the amount of fluid is not related to orgasmic pleasure. Rather than feeling pressure to perform in any way, focus on your unique experience and relish in every erotic moment.

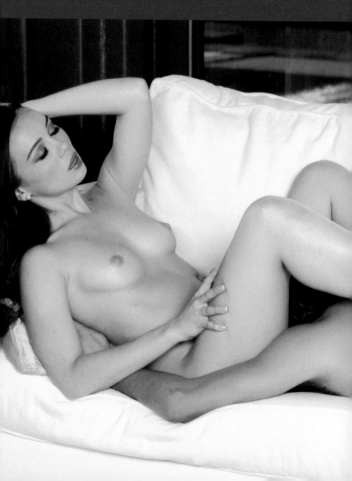

Hart's line is the pathway that surrounds the super sensitive vestibule of her sweet vulva. This is the shiny section between her inner lips and is the site of the glands associated with lubrication and female ejaculation. Trace lusty licks around this sensitive area to deepen your connection and unleash a storm of sensuality from between her legs.

THE BASICS

- Use your tongue to trace a sweet path over Hart's line as you tease her body to the heights of orgasmic pleasure.
- Send her body into a tsunami of sexual pleasure by using a small vibrator to trace Hart's line while sliding two crossed fingers in and out of her vagina.

LICK BY LICK

- Lower the lights and approach her from behind while she's watching television or sitting at the table.
- Wrap your arms around her and kiss her neck before moving on to her lips. Kneel at her feet.
- Slide her bum to the edge of the chair or couch and undress her from the waist down before spreading her legs.
- Use the backs of your fingers to very gently trace curvy lines over her inner thighs to draw blood flow and awareness to the area.
- Gently peel open her inner labia with your thumbs and use a flat tongue to lick the shiny vestibule from bottom to top as slowly as possible.
- Twirl your tongue around her fourchette (the delicate spot at the bottom of where her labia meet).
- When she starts moaning and squirming with delight, finish her off by tracing the tip of your tongue around the outer edge of her vestibule. Alternate between clockwise and counterclockwise rotations, maintaining a rapid, steady rhythm.

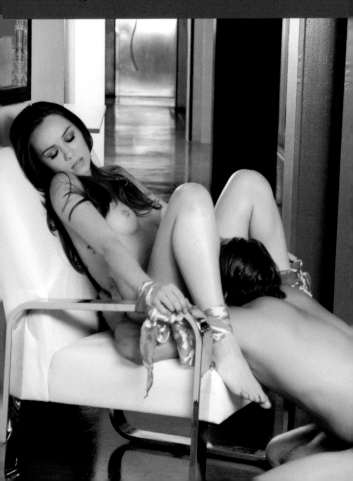

Although orgasm-inducing finishing moves are always welcome, sometimes a little denial can be just what she needs to truly appreciate your expert oral skills.

THE BASICS

- Tie her down and tease her entire body until she's pleading for your orgasmic touch.

- The hottest sex is in your head, not between your legs. Sexual teasing can be even more intoxicating than direct genital touch, as it allows your imagination to run wild with erotic anticipation. To eroticize your relationship be playful and tease your lover throughout the day with sexy compliments and flirtatious sexual references.

LICK BY LICK

- With her advanced consent, tie her wrists and ankles to the bed posts or chair legs using silk scarves.

- Ask her where she likes to be touched and then tease the area all around this craving erogenous zone without actually touching it. Breathe over it with warm air, getting as close as you can without making physical contact.

- Do the same to her sweet vulva: trickle your fingers around it; press your lips into her thighs, allowing your cheeks to brush up against her labia only fleetingly; lick her *mons* and twirl your tongue over her clitoral hood as lightly as possible.

- Add a few fingers to the game as you pet her pussy, but when she starts to get really riled up, retreat to kissing her neck.

- Repeat this teasing sequence a few times, encouraging her to tell you just how badly she craves it.

- Once her body is straining with near-orgasmic pleasure, dive in with your lips, tongue, and fingers, and give it to her just how she likes it.

- When you're done, be sure to tell her teasingly, "You're welcome."

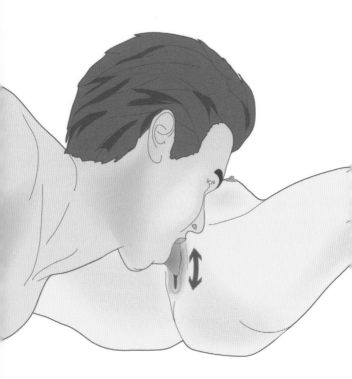

Under the Hood allows you to stroke and stimulate the super sensitive clitoral shaft and head even once it retracts under the hood, making it an indispensable technique for every skilled lover.

THE BASICS

- Use your tongue to slide the hood of her clitoris over its shaft and swollen head.

- If her vulva becomes too slippery, you may not be able to manipulate her hood with your tongue. If this is the case, simply use your thumbs to glide it back and forth while sliding your tongue inside her vagina.

LICK BY LICK

- Take total control for this move and bend her over a chair, table, bed, or couch.

- Separate her legs with your hands and suck her inner labia from behind while twirling your tongue between them.

- Sit down on the ground beneath her and pull her body a few inches out from the furniture so that you can slide your head between her legs. Turn around so you're facing her.

- Twist your tongue around the inner wall of her vagina and slide a wet thumb between her butt cheeks to periodically tease her pucker.

- When her hips start to thrust consistently, take her over the edge by sliding her hood back and forth over her shaft and head using the tip of your tongue.

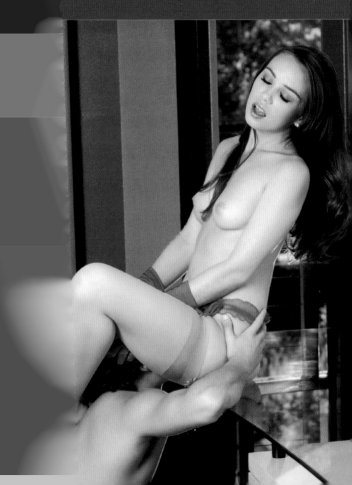

Venturing down between her legs is a powerful act that balances power, vulnerability, trust, and intimacy. Intensify the experience by letting her take the reins of control as you work your magic with your expert tongue.

THE BASICS

She wraps her feet around the back of your neck and uses them to guide you both to the heights of passion and pleasure.

LICK BY LICK

- Play with power by laying her on the bed and telling her that you want to ravage her luscious body.

- Lie between her legs and wrap her feet and ankles behind your neck.

- Look up into her eyes and tell her to show you how she likes it.

- Press your tongue flat against her pussy and moan a little to create vibrations. Let her guide your pressure, movements, and speed with her legs.

- Make lots of noise to show appreciation for her pussy.

- If you can reach her breasts, wrap your fingers around them and have her place her hands on top to control your caresses.

- When she comes, tell her how much you love it, and keep licking her pussy even after her orgasm subsides.

- Pay close attention to the guidance of her legs and hip movements. If she's thrusting into you, you've probably found a sweet spot, so don't stop what you're doing. Variety may be the spice of life, but when it comes to toe-curling orgasms, switching back and forth between moves at the peak of pleasure can cause more frustration than frenzy.

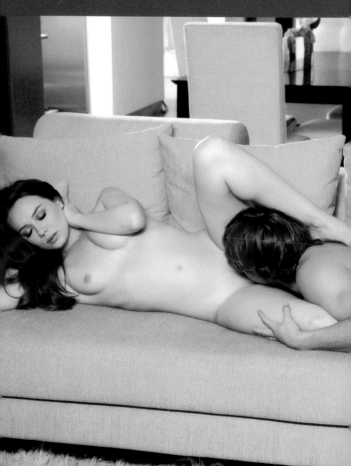

Are you an expert at going down? Would you consider yourself a connoisseur of eating the peach? Show her just how much you love to taste, lick, and suck on her sweetest parts by accentuating your slurps, kisses, and moans. Your enthusiasm will not only put her at ease, but her relaxation can encourage orgasmic response.

THE BASICS
Bury your face in her pussy and suck on it like you're eating a peach—minus the teeth.

LICK BY LICK

• Tell her how much you love her pussy and how sweet it tastes in your mouth.

• Climb between her legs as she lies on her side and you lie facing her.

• Wrap your lips around the outer edges of her vulva as though you're biting into the juiciest peach with your lips covering your teeth.

• Suck away, tasting every last drop and allowing the juices to drip down your face.

• Pay attention to her sounds, and accentuate your own moans as she lets out indulgent squeals of gratification.

• Grab hold off her butt cheeks with both hands and press her body into your face as you tell her she's delicious.

• When her body reaches a pinnacle of pleasure, bury your tongue in her vagina as you continue sucking with your wet, soft lips.

• Hot sex is messy, slippery, and even a bit slimy, so don't be shy about getting her juices all over your face. And if she's hesitant to let you press your entire face into her pussy, ply her with compliments (on a regular basis—not just during sex) to support a positive body image that includes her genitals.

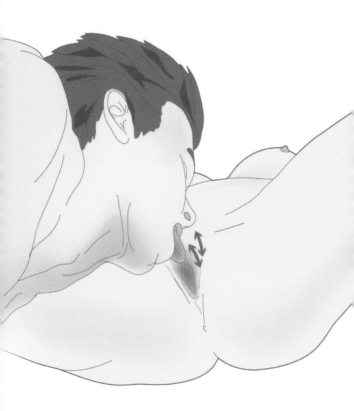

Combine different strokes, licks, angles, and patterns to keep her guessing all night long. Even when you find a combo that makes her moan, don't stop there, as her body's unique responses change daily, setting the scene for a lifetime of erotic discovery.

THE BASICS

- Vary your tongue strokes and licks to gauge her response. Once she's close to going over the edge, launch her into a sexual trance by picking her favorite move of the day and increasing the speed and pressure.

- Change positions and try the same techniques from different angles to vary the sensations.

LICK BY LICK

Begin with some basic tongue screwing, then vary your tongue movements to include:

- Wide circles tracing the inside of her vaginal walls.

- Sweeping figure eights over her labia.

- A curled-up tongue against her swollen G-spot on the upper wall of her vagina.

- A wide V-shaped stroke over the entire vulva.

- Deep insertion with your tongue rolled up into a tight tube.

- Side-to-side motions just inside the vagina, where most of the responsive nerve endings are located.

- Gentle pulses over her sensitive clitoral head.

- Passionate flicks over her fourchette (the lowest point where her labia meet) followed by wide upward strokes with a flat tongue.

- Winding "S" strokes up her thighs and over her vaginal opening.

- Very gentle nibbling of her inner labia.

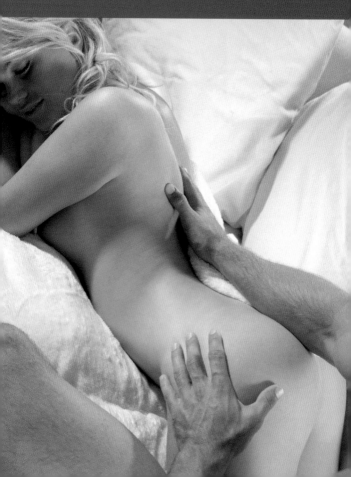

AH, THERE'S THE RUB

Rubbing-off is many a lady's favorite pastime, as it's a reliable way to reach orgasm with intensity and speed. Women often lie on their stomachs and use a vibrator, bed sheet, pillow, or hand to rub themselves into a sexual oblivion. Combine her go-to self-stimulation move with the warmth and intimacy of your touch, and you've got a recipe for ecstasy.

THE BASICS

Slide your tongue and fingers beneath her as she teaches you her unique rubbing-off technique.

LICK BY LICK

- Have her lie on her stomach, as this position allows her to create extra friction using her bodyweight against her sensitive mons and clitoris.

- Straddle her lower back facing her feet and offer a sensuous back rub to help get you both into the mood.

- Once you're both feeling relaxed, slide one hand under her pelvis.

- She can reach down and place her hand on yours to steer the rubbing motion. She'll also control the pressure and amount of friction by adjusting the weight of her body against your hand.

- Once she finds her rhythm, start stroking your cock with your other hand in perfect rhythm with her passionate rubbing.

- Lube and orgasms usually go hand-in-hand, but rubbing orgasms may be the exception depending on your lover's unique tastes. Because you'll be rubbing her mons and vulva without penetration, too much lube may inhibit the friction needed for this particular technique, so check in with her to ascertain just how wet she wants it.

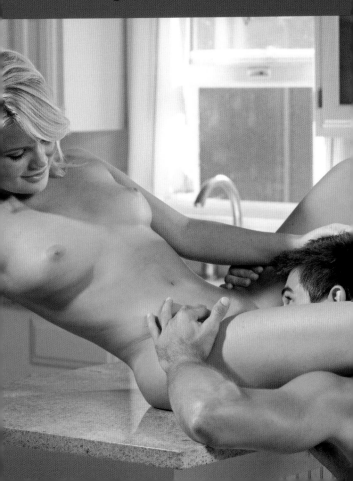

Make her purr as you lap up everything her juicy pussy has to offer. Your quick, consistent tongue strokes will make her quiver with delight and prolong her arousal, carrying her from one orgasm to the next.

THE BASICS

- Use your tongue to lick her from bottom to top as though you're lapping up water from a bowl.

- As she approaches orgasm, her clitoris may become too sensitive to handle your tongue's licks, so be aware of her reactions and adjust your pressure and positioning accordingly. Besides, focusing solely on her clit while ignoring the rest of her beautiful lady parts is comparable to sucking *only* the head of a man's penis during a blow job.

LICK BY LICK

- Have her lean against the headboard with her legs bent and feet flat on the mattress.

- Prop her hips up with a few pillows to ensure easier access to her juiciest parts.

- Tuck your head between her thighs and curl your tongue into the very bottom of her vulva, licking in a scooping motion, as though you're drinking water from a bowl.

- Begin with slow, steady licks and work your way up to her *mons*.

- As her arousal levels increase, speed up your licks until your tongue is fervently lapping up her juices with several licks per second.

- As she comes, lower your tongue to the center of her vulva and keep licking away. If it's too much for her to take, retreat to her thighs or perineum, but don't let her get away with one orgasm alone. Give her a few moments to regroup before building up the tongue-induced storm of sensuality once again.

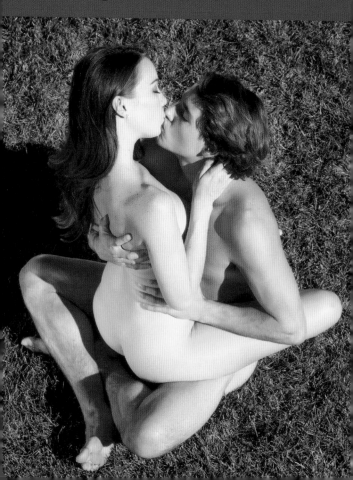

A kiss is one of the most sensual physical acts. As your lips meet, a flurry of sexual energy erupts in the brain and throughout the body. It goes without saying that oral sex creates an even more impassioned reaction, making *The French Kiss* the perfect move that balances both carnal lust and deep connection.

THE BASICS

- Kiss her vulva as though you're giving it a passionate French kiss!
- Pepper your day with unexpected kisses to set the mood and leave her wanting more. And make kissing a daily habit, as science suggests that men can actually transfer small doses of testosterone to their lover through a prolonged French kiss. Higher levels of testosterone are associated with increased libido.

LICK BY LICK

- Kiss her passionately on the lips to give her a taste of what's to come.
- Continue to build the sexual tension by caressing her legs, alternating between your gentle fingertips and the warm, firm palms of your hand.
- Take a deep breath and exhale over her pussy before making contact to fuel her anticipation.
- Trace wide ovals over her vulva with a soft tongue and feather-light touch.
- Stick your tongue out and point it downward, pressing the entire surface against her lips. Sweep your tongue from side to side like the pendulum of a grandfather clock.
- Dive in with your lips and tongue and French kiss her pussy with your lips, tongue, and face. Show your enthusiasm with your sounds and breath, and don't be afraid to get a bit messy.

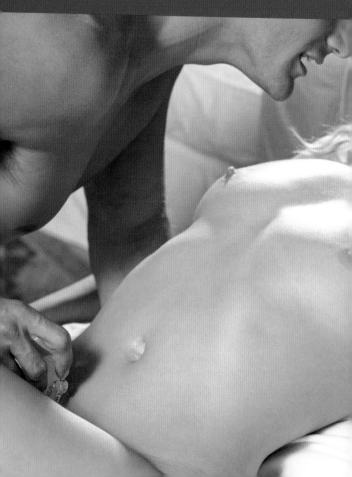

Playing with temperature is a pro-secret for mind-blowing oral sex, as the tingly sensations of hot and cold undoubtedly intensify your sexual response.

THE BASICS

- Set a glass of ice water and a mug of peppermint tea at your bedside, and keep your lover guessing as you change up the pace and turn up the heat.

- Add a little amaretto, rum, or bourbon to your mint tea, or use a mint-flavored breath strip to heighten the tingle.

LICK BY LICK

- Begin by breathing warm and cool air over her pussy without making physical contact with your mouth. A wide open mouth will create a warm sensation, while tight pursed lips will generate cooler air.

- Take a sip of the water and tuck a small ice cube into your cheek as you begin licking, sucking, and kissing her labia. Don't place the ice cube directly on her skin, but allow the ice to cool your lips, tongue, and inner cheeks.

- After a minute or two, heat things up by taking a sip of the hot tea before you dive back in and resume your slurping, smooching, and stroking. Keep sipping periodically to maintain the heat and breathe over the wet spots to make them quiver with delight!

- If you're going to add your hands into the mix, dip them in the cool water before playing with your lover's nipples or running a few fingers over her backside.

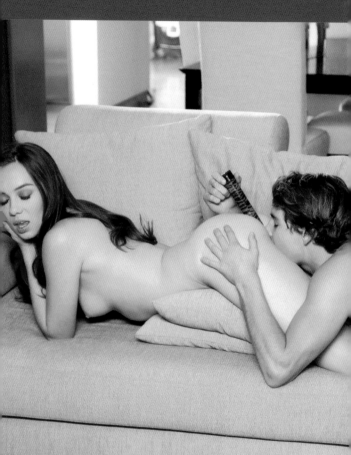

If you want to share the erotic sensations of anal play without penetrating the pucker, we've got good news for you! The lower vagina actually shares a common wall with the anus, so you can double her delight by pleasuring the pussy and bum simultaneously.

THE BASICS

- Use a finger, toy, or tongue to simulate anal play through the lower vaginal wall.
- When she's about to come, keep stimulating the shared vaginal-anal wall and slide another finger into her wet pussy, pressing downward toward her stomach to caress her G-spot.

LICK BY LICK

- Straddle her at the knees while she lies on her stomach atop a pile of pillows.
- Tease your lover with kisses over her soft butt cheeks, and kiss the top of the slit between them without diving in.
- Separate her legs and fondle her inner thighs with both hands. Tell her how much you like the view from behind.
- Slide your hands below her hips and lick the sides of her pussy from front to back, separating her inner lips slowly and sensually.
- Push your lips out into a large oval shape and suck her into your mouth before inserting your tongue.
- Slide your tongue in and out, curling it up toward her bum at the deepest point of penetration. As you lick her, use your hands against her hips to thrust her into your face.
- If she wants more depth or pressure, use your fingers or a toy to curl up in a 'come hither' motion against the back wall of her vagina. Remember that since she's lying on her stomach, you want to curl upward toward her bum.

© 2015 Quarto Publishing Group USA Inc.
Text © 2013 Jessica O'Reilly
Photography © 2013 Quiver

First published in 2015 by Quiver,
an imprint of The Quarto Group,
100 Cummings Center, Suite 265-D,
Beverly, MA 01915, USA.
T (978) 282-9590 F (978) 283-2742
www.QuartoKnows.com

Quiver titles are also available at discount for retail, wholesale, promotional, and bulk purchase. For details, contact the Special Sales Manager by email at specialsales@quarto.com or by mail at The Quarto Group, Attn: Special Sales Manager, 100 Cummings Center, Suite 265-D, Beverly, MA 01915, USA.

The Publisher maintains the records relating to images in this book required by 18 USC 2257. Records are located at The Quarto Group, 100 Cummings Center, Suite 265-D, Beverly, MA 01915, USA.

20   14 15

ISBN: 978-59233-665-4

Library of Congress Cataloging-in-Publication Data available

Cover design by traffic
Photography by Richard Avery and Holly Randall
Illustrations by Robert Brandt

Printed and bound in Hong Kong